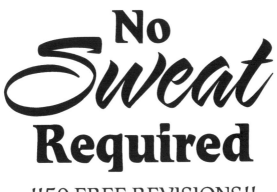

No
Sweat
Required

!!50 FREE REVISIONS!!

MICHELLE FAY

authorHOUSE®

AuthorHouse™
1663 Liberty Drive
Bloomington, IN 47403
www.authorhouse.com
Phone: 1 (800) 839-8640

Published by AuthorHouse 12/07/2016

ISBN: 978-1-5246-5141-1 (sc)
ISBN: 978-1-5246-5140-4 (e)

Library of Congress Control Number: 2016919502

Print information available on the last page.

Any people depicted in stock imagery provided by Thinkstock are models, and such images are being used for illustrative purposes only. Certain stock imagery © Thinkstock.

This book is printed on acid-free paper.

Contents

This book was written for the sole purpose of helping people like me, who have battled with their weight. All information in this book is based on my own personal experience with my desire to lose weight and become healthy!

When I started "my program," as I call it, I weighed 180 pounds, and at five-foot-four, I was slowly killing myself. My body mass was thirty-one, but with the use my program, I now weigh 130 pounds, and my body mass is twenty-two. It feels great to have lost fifty pounds. I thank God every day for blessing me with the strength and knowledge to lose the weight. Praying to Him for help with weight loss was my very first step. He answered my prayer and guided me all the way and still does to this day! I couldn't have done it without Him.

My biggest thanks go out to my OB-GYN and my family doctor, who supported me all the way. Because I had been having some problems, I went to see her. Her news was that the weight on my lower body had caused my uterus to drop. She said, "You need a *hysterectomy!*" I almost fainted! I mean I felt fine, just some pain in my lower body. I felt beautiful even with the extra weight. I really had not thought about the extra weight. It was just easier to keep eating and not worry about the fact that I had put on an extra fifty pounds in the last four to five years. I mean, I was a busy person, trying to raise four children, build a home, stay married in today's world, and just be happy, but I was slowing killing myself! I was eating the wrong things and eating triple the portions. I quickly learned that a fifteen-dollar food scale could show me the right portion, even if I was still eating the wrong foods.

Hey, it was a start, and I had to start somewhere, right? But once I got the portions in my head for one person instead of three, I remembered, "No more eating for three people!"

It was all starting to come together.

The food scale became my best friend for two weeks. It jump-started my thinking about food and just how much I was consuming. So please try to invest in a food scale to curb your eating habits for your own sake.

After three months of doing this program, my OB-GYN was amazed! My uterus was starting to shift back to the place where it belonged in my body! That was a year and a half ago, and I did not have to have a hysterectomy! I no longer had to fight with the fat and extra weight. Thank God! I know this is all a little personal, but I believe this program is what saved my life. If my OB-GYN had never told me that I would need to have a hysterectomy, I would still be overweight and probably sick by now. I was thirty-two years old at the time. I felt I was too young to have such a major surgery … and all because I was eating myself to death!

I hope that in this book, you'll find success like I did!

I started my program on April 21, 2009, a Tuesday, but it's not important when you start. The important thing is that you *start*. I weighed 180 pounds. I now weigh 130 pounds. I wore a size fourteen. I now wear a size four! I never really thought I would lose those fifty pounds! But I did! And you can too! It feels so good to feel good again! I was so used to feeling bad that I had forgotten what good felt like, but not anymore.

I also did my food journal for six months, but it has been a year and a half since I started my program! With my program, I lost seven to eight pounds a month. That's a healthy way to lose weight, because if you lose too much too fast, you're only going to gain it back again and possibly double the weight. It's not all about the number on the scale. It's about how you feel once you see the numbers going down, and believe me, when you see those numbers dropping, you'll want to keep going, because you're going to feel better and look better. You can do this!

Chapter 1

Calorie Intake

Calorie intake is very important, but at the same time, it's quite simple to manage with a little knowledge. It's really simple math. After speaking with my doctor, I learned that the human body burns an average of two thousand calories a day, no matter what we do. So even if we choose to sit and do absolutely nothing, our body burns at least those two thousand calories.

So, if you only took five hundred calories from your diet per day, you would have lost four pounds in one month. "Why?" you ask. Simple: because your body is still burning two thousand calories a day. But you have not reduced yours to 1,500 calories a day. Congratulations! You've burned five hundred calories, and you aren't even sweating yet!

Now that we have learned that part of the math problem, you can learn how to count calories the easy and fun way. One simple way to do this is to read the labels, use your food scale, measure the portions, and then write down what you have eaten. This is what I did!

A lot of products contain more than one serving of food, but because we are hungry consumers, we fail to think about how much we have just eaten. Because of that, we gain weight. In this chapter, I present a few examples of food labels so that you can better understand this process.

Look at the serving size first and then measure out the correct size portion and finally write down the calorie information. Measure your food for at least two weeks. This will help you learn your serving sizes and calorie information for the foods you eat on a regular basis. On average, the consumer eats the same foods over and over every two weeks. We just mix up the days that we eat our meals. Once you start writing down what you eat, you, too, will see this pattern. It's kind of neat to look back and see the patterns.

We now must learn to write down what we have eaten for the day. The simplest way to do this is to grab a pen and notebook and start writing. I myself used a wonderful book that I purchased online just for this reason. It was the best tool of all, besides the pen, of course! I do believe I used three books. After the first week, it was just another part of my day. I did this for about six months. It is actually quite fascinating to look back on what I had eaten compared to what I eat now, because now I feel and look wonderful! In the back of this book, you'll find a thirty-day food journal to help you get started.

Now, we have the label-reading down. You're probably wondering, "Hey, what if I go out to eat?" Personally, I eat out a lot just like most people in the United States today. Calorie information was not something I could find quickly at my local drive-through, but I quickly learned that almost every major restaurant has calorie information online. Thank God for the person who started that idea! Now I just had to find the time to look up where and what I ate. But with four kids, a husband, a house to maintain, laundry, and don't forget cooking (sometimes), who has the time? However, we all have ten seconds to spare to go online and check the calories at a restaurant. You can do what I did and check out those calories and serving sizes from your favorite places to eat. You'll be amazed at what you have eaten. I know that I was! But don't feel guilty. Just try again tomorrow. Believe me, you will remember those numbers. And with each day, you will remember even more numbers. Just don't get scared. Remember that these *are only numbers.* Just keep writing them down! Also, for the fun of it, you can throw in your feelings for the day or what's going on in your busy life. Just keep writing the information down! In the back of this book, you'll also find ten major restaurants with their calorie information. This will help you get started with the dining-out problem.

Bottom Line Numbers that Equal Success

For women, that number is 1,500 calories a day.
For men, that number is 1,800 calories a day.

Remember: for every 500 calories you don't eat each day, that equals a grand total of 3,500 calories after a whole week.
Yes, I'm saying that you can lose weight with fewer calories. One week equals one to a half of a pound lighter. Yippee! You did it! Sweating yet? Keep writing.

In one month, you can lose four to six pounds.
In two months, you could have lost up to twelve pounds.

Keep writing; it gets better with each entry into your food journal.

Tips for Reading Food Labels

Read labels to compare key ingredients, and make smart choices to improve your nutritional habits. Use the following sample food label and diagram to sharpen your label-reading skills:

Ingredients: These are listed by weight, the most to the least.

- Limit products where fats and sugars appear early in the list.
- Limit products containing "shortening" or "partially hydrogenated" fats.
- Limit products containing coconut, palm oil, cocoa butter, butter, or lard.

Serving size: All the nutritional numbers listed in this section are based on the "severing size" amount. Compare the serving size to the amount you eat. For example, if you ate two cups of this food, you'd double the numbers shown, because a serving for this food is one cup.

Servings per container: Even small packages sometimes contain more than one serving.

Total fat: Low-fat foods contain three grams or less of fat per serving.

Saturated fat: This raises blood cholesterol levels. Food low in saturated fat contains less than 0.5 grams of saturated fat per serving.

Trans fat: Trans fats result from adding hydrogen to vegetable oils. Look for "hydrogenated" oils in the ingredient list to know if a food contains trans fat.

- Cookies, crackers, French fries, donuts, and other commercial fried and baked foods are major sources of trans fat in the diet.
- Trans fat raises the LDL (bad) cholesterol and lowers the HDL (good) cholesterol.
- Limit your intake of saturated fat and trans fat to less than 10 percent of total calories.
- The Food and Drug Administration (FDA) requires food manufacturers list trans fat on food labels.

Cholesterol: This is found only in animal foods. It is recommended that you eat less than 200 milligrams of cholesterol per day.

Sodium: This is the part of salt that can raise blood pressure and cause fluid retention. Good choices contain 400 milligrams or less per serving.

Total carbohydrate: This is a total that includes starches, sugars, and fiber.

Portion Size Comparison

A small milk carton equals about 1 cup (8 oz) of milk or yogurt

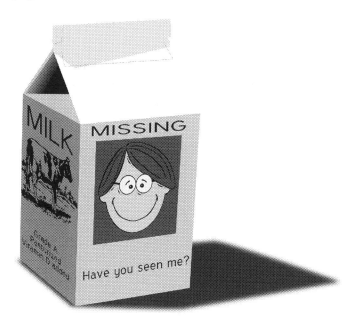

A tennis ball is a serving of fruit or vegetables

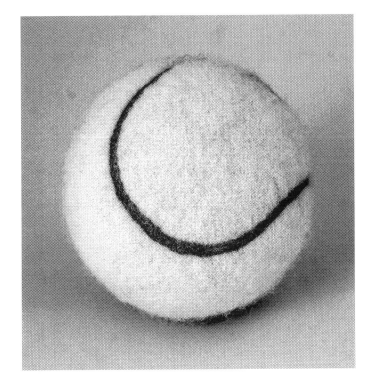

A bar of soap or a full deck of cards is about 3 ounces of meat, poultry, or fish

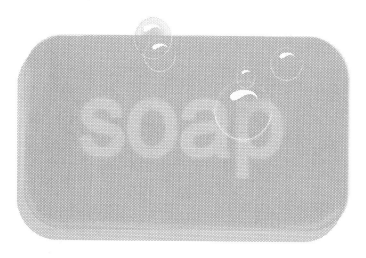

or

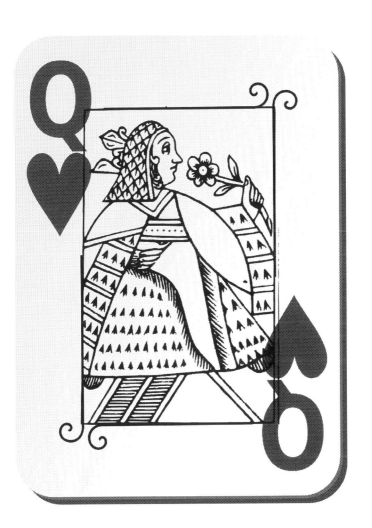

2 cassette tapes equal 2 slices of bread

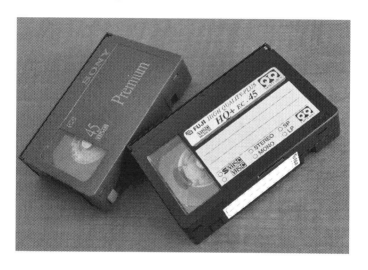

2 quarters equal about 2 tablespoons of peanut butter

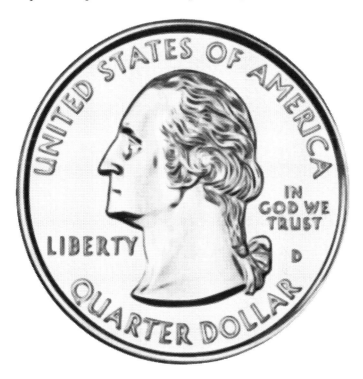

1 penny equals about 1 teaspoon of oil, mayonnaise, margarine or butter

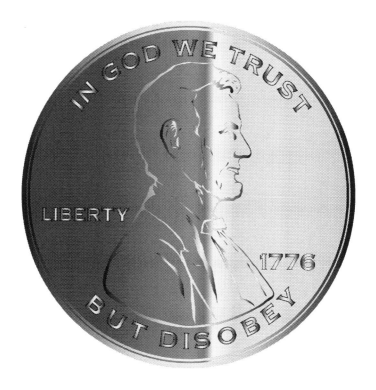

A computer mouse is about the same size as one medium potato

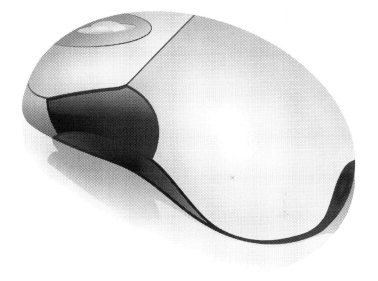

4 dice equal a one-ounce serving of cheese

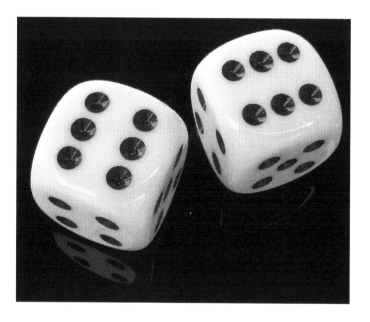

Chapter 2

B-12 Intake

Vitamin B-12 plays an important role in body function. It helps with many things. For me, B-12 gave me the energy to do a little more each day. This was wonderful because I didn't feel tired or stressed out! When I first learned about the benefits of B-12 in helping with weight loss, I was completely shocked, because I had thought, *Hey, don't I get enough of that already?* Well, I came to find out that most of us could use a little extra B-12. The main source of B-12 comes from red meat, which I don't really eat a lot of. So once again, I went on the Internet and found out that I could buy a one-month supply of B-12 shots for three hundred dollars, liquid gold, and I willingly paid! Weight loss—I wanted it badly, and the companies knew this. Just think of all the fad diets, pills, and whatever else is out there. A very scary thought!

However, this three-hundred-dollar liquid gold did in fact help me! I felt wonderful. Having energy was great! Therefore, I kept busy. I felt relaxed and even slept better. The only catch was that I didn't have three hundred dollars for B-12 shots every month. So what could I do? I called my doctor and made an appointment just to talk about this problem.

He was great. He explained the B-12 shots to me. He also agreed that the B-12 shots that I had ordered had in fact helped me. So he gave me a prescription for B-12 shots that I could give myself at home, which meant no more three hundred dollars a month for B-12! I could now give myself the shot at home twice a week for around twenty-four dollars a month. B-12 shots are normally given to older people who have very little energy, but my doctor understood just how much these shots really were helping me. I was so scared during the first one my husband gave me. I think I scared him! After that, the B-12 shots just became another part of my weekly routine. Life wasn't so crazy now. At least it seemed that way, and it was true! I felt amazing! I started going for walks with my family, having fun, and burning a few calories at the same time! It was great to feel good again!

I did the B-12 shots for about three months. After that time period, I was good to go and still going. I just needed the B-12 shots to establish a good routine. Sometimes I still give myself a B-12 shot, but it's rare now that I've lost fifty pounds! I don't feel as if I need them as much anymore. No more sticking myself, although the tiny pain was well worth the results.

I chose the shot because after lots of research and my doctor's final approval, I just felt that the shot was the best for me. The first month, I did the shots twice a week. Then during the second month, I only did the shot once a week. By the third month, I only did the shot every other week. Talk to your doctor today! Why wait any longer for your weight-loss dream to come true?

Chapter 3

Water Intake

The amount of water that I try very hard to drink is about two liters per day. It sounds like a lot of water to consume in one day, but it's really not. For me, the best way to do this was to buy one-liter containers with sports caps and carry them with me. Another thing that I chose to do was buy bottled water and have one with me wherever I go, even in the bathroom! It worked, and it has become yet another part of my daily routine. I still haven't sweated yet. The process is really quite simple. Just drink water, and drink of lot of it. You will be amazed at how wonderful water can make you feel, not only on the inside but the outside as well.

The Beauty of Nature Comes from Water!

I know that I've made everything sound really simple, but truth be told, it's hard. We are told every day to drink water with *sugar*. For me, giving up sugar meant (no energy). That was not cool. I needed all the energy I could get (just not that kind of energy)! That's where the B-12 shots came in. Now I no longer needed the sugar! I thought giving up my sweet tea was going to kill me, but now I have my unsweetened tea with lots of lemons to save the day! Or there are the days when half sweetened and half unsweetened might just have to save the day! I still eat and drink the things I love. I just try to mentally keep track of the calories I've consumed. I do enjoy life's sweetness, but I try not to go overboard.

I do indulge myself! Dark chocolate is my pitfall, especially if it has almonds! Both are very good for you in limited amounts.

Life's too short! Just don't forget to drink your water!

Chapter 4

Fiber Intake and Detoxing the Body

Who knew getting one's fiber could be so easy? Forget that tired, old bowl of oatmeal. There's new oatmeal bars in all kinds of flavors that are loaded with fiber! Some bars have up to twelve grams of fiber in just one bar.

Here are just a few brands that I chose to eat:

1. Kashi products (local grocery store).
2. Fiber One products (local grocery store).
3. VitaTop muffins: Mint chocolate is my favorite, and they also have only a hundred calories and six grams of fiber per muffin (local grocery and online).
4. Fiber Gourmet products (online): They have pasta and snack crackers (fourteen grams of fiber).

5. Lori's Earth Friendly Products (online): The juice boxes have ten grams of fiber (apple, orange, and grape).

6. Barilla Products: These are great too (local grocery store).

All of these products taste wonderful and have a lot of health benefits aside from the fiber in them. My kids have even found their favorite ones. Imagine that! I've not only helped myself but my children as well. That's a wonderful feeling all by itself!

And hopefully this information will help you as well.

My personal goal for fiber intake is at least thirty-five grams a day. It was really easy with all the wonderful food that I chose. Your fiber intake usually goes by your age. For me, the chart said twenty-five to thirty grams, but I feel better with at least thirty-five grams a day. So you should judge how your body reacts to adding more fiber and see what your number is. I was thirty-three when I started adding more fiber, so go ahead and try to add more fiber to your diet, and then you can feel and see the wonderful benefits of fiber! It's almost an instant tummy tuck without the scar!

Detoxing the Body

The outside of our body is like a gigantic walking sponge. Everything we eat, drink, and breathe is absorbed into our organs. Over time, all of this stuff builds up in our bodies. We get rid of some of it by sweating, bathing, and of course, going to the bathroom. But we never really get rid of all of it. The inside of our body is like a car. I mean, you wouldn't keep driving your car without changing the oil, right? You know that it will eventually break down from the sludge buildup. Our bodies will do the same. That's why detoxing your body is so important! I tried so many products for detoxifying the body that it's not even funny.

But only one product worked. The name of this wonderful product is Dr. Natura's Whole Body Cleanse. If you have never done a whole-body cleanse, I highly recommend this product. For first-time people, the company recommends three months and then a yearly one-month cleanse after that. I personally did both the three-month and the yearly one-month cleanses. The results were amazing! The things that build up in our bodies look very scary, but I'm glad they're gone. The cleanse makes you feel like you have a new body, inside and out. Once again, the results are amazing! Just try it out for yourself.

Also, instead of joining the gym for their equipment, go for the sauna. Saunas are great at cleansing the build of everyday pollutants, such as heavy metals and the chemicals found in what we drink and eat. All of this builds up, and the sauna, especially the infrared saunas, goes down to the bone marrow and helps the body release all these toxicants. It'll help with skin, hair, and a lot of different health issues. Being in a sauna can help you burn around three hundred calories in a thirty- to forty-minute session, depending on the heat setting. Saunas can range in price from three hundred to ten thousand dollars. If you have the cash to spare, buy one for your home. After a hard day at work, relax in it and then sleep like a baby and wake up feeling refreshed and ready to conquer the world! Another great tool is a steam shower loaded with essential oils. Steam showers make you sweat while you are showering, but they add the health benefits of the essential oils. For centuries, people have used oils for their healing powers. A steam shower can cost anywhere from three hundred to a thousand dollars, depending on what you want. Steam showers don't go as deep into your body as saunas do, but they have their place in health, too. They're great for kids with colds or allergies. Add a little eucalyptus oil, and they're back to breathing normal again. It helps them relax after a hard day and sleep better at night. You are also teaching them to care about their health and adopt behaviors that will improve their health naturally.

This may all sound like a lot of money, but just think of how much you have already wasted on fad diets, diet pills, special foods, and equipment, not to mention all that gas and babysitting money and your time running to the gym. That may be what you like to do, but for me, it wasn't. I enjoy a nice, relaxing steam shower at home with a little lavender oil and then heading to bed, not getting the kids from the daycare and then driving home and putting the kids to bed. After that, I'm stressed out again! Now I just put my kids to bed and really enjoy that steam shower. It's my little bliss in life!

Between the sauna (which was a Mother's Day gift), a steam shower, and the gazelle (which was a Christmas present), the total spent over two years was $2,500.00. But all this is mine, not the local gym's. My equipment has already paid for itself. I've lost weight! I'm healthier, and I feel amazing! Plus, my kids get to enjoy all of this as well. At the gym, that's a no-no.

You've heard it before: "Eat your veggies and all of them!" I'm not going to give you a long, drawn-out chapter about why you should, because you already know why. But I am going to give you a friendly reminder. Just eat your veggies! Your mother would be proud, and you'll increase your fiber intake at the same time. Plus, veggies are low in calories. If you're like me though and you just feel like you don't have the time, buy the precut, prewashed, and prepackaged ones! Carry them in your car or take them to work. Veggies are excellent raw, and they give you more fiber too! At restaurants, order doubles of your favorite kinds! Please just eat your veggies! You'll be glad you did!

Look at the photos above. Thought you were hungry? Think again! Your friends are the hungry ones. They are the ones craving the sugar and carbs. That's what they need to reproduce! And guess what happens when they do? Your belly aches and grows just a little bigger. This is to accommodate more friends! This may sound weird, disgusting, and unbelievable, but it's true! So, unless you like these kinds of friends, start your cleanse today! And say *good-bye* to your not-so-good friends forever!

Chapter 5

Exercise Output

For me, I thought that this would be the hardest part of all, but I came to find out that it was the most exciting part! You can burn calories doing just about anything. It's absolutely amazing! I found all kinds of ways to burn calories, including cleaning those toilets. This is not fun by the way, but it's necessary at times! No live-in maid for this mommy.

Once again, the person who invented the Internet saved me time. I looked up every exercise possible. Naturally, sex was the one that interested me the most. Sounds bad, I know, but sex is part of a healthy and loving relationship, which I have with my husband of fifteen years. So that's what I chose.

It may sound kind of bad; however, burning calories was important to me, and having sex is fun (at least for me it is). I had found the perfect exercise for me. Sex also increases a chemical called oxytocin, which is your "cuddle hormone" and which helps with bonding, reduces fear, and stimulates endorphins. So, ladies and gentlemen, go for it! Let those endorphins take away the pain. After orgasm, your dopamine levels fall; however, your prolactin levels rise, and both partners have that relaxed feeling or that sleepy feeling that most men get. A study done at Duke University found that women who enjoyed sex lived seven to eight years longer than women who didn't and that men lived longer as well. Another study done in 1989 in France found that women who had sex and enjoyed it at least three times a week were less likely to develop breast cancer, but the biological mechanism is unclear. Either way, I enjoy having sex with my husband, and if it helps me live seven to eight years longer and have better moods and less pain, then I'm all for it. In 2002, another study done at the University of New York found that women who had sex and enjoyed it had better moods and had less depression problems than women who didn't have sex. The reason that happens is because the semen contains testosterone, estrogen, prolactin, and prostaglandins, which passes through the vaginal walls into the bloodstream and makes us happier. I don't know about you, but I need all the happy hormones I can get!

Who knew burning calories could be so much fun. Every position has a different potential for the amount of calories that you can burn! This was my kind of exercise, and as I lost weight, sex became even more enjoyable than before.

It felt as though ten years had dropped off of my body. I'm not sure where it went, and I don't really care. I'm just glad it's gone!

All jokes aside, it really did work, but I'm sure it had more to do with the breathing exercises that I did while I was having sex. I did deep breathing, inhaling through my nose and then slowly exhaling through my mouth. This activity is great for your heart and lungs. It's sort of like yoga, just not solo. Add an exercise ball for fun. Consider practicing yoga, and then watch your body transform. Doing yoga as a couple can stimulate sexy feelings, which can lead to fun inside and outside the bedroom.

I'm not trying to say that you shouldn't exercise in the traditional way. I'm just trying to give new meaning to the word exercise. Besides sex, breathing is my first choice of exercise.

My second favorite one was Tony Little's Gazelle, which is an awesome machine! It burns tons of calories and shapes your body at the same time. I used this quite often, about two or three times a week. The first couple of weeks, I worked out for about ten minutes three times a week.

Once I built up more energy and saw the pounds disappearing, I would typically stay on the machine for about an hour, which would burn around eight to nine hundred calories. Once again, this was an awesome machine!

My third favorite way to burn those calories was walking with a shoe called FitFlop. FitFlop shoes are designed to help build muscles in your lower body. And they do! They are another wonderful tool. I now own three pairs of FitFlop shoes. I wear them three times a week, whether I'm cleaning house, taking walks, or grocery shopping.

However you chose to get your exercise, it is your choice. Just remember to try to have fun with it! Some days, it will be easy to get those extra calories burned, and other days, it won't be so easy! Just don't beat yourself up about it. Try again tomorrow, even if it's only for ten minutes.

Better than Zero Minutes!

Another great thing to do is stretch as often as possible. Personally, I love stretching in the shower and using a doorframe to pull myself up and really stretch my arms out. You can also use the doorframe to push yourself forward, and this stretches the back part of your arms. I always find it's best to stretch first thing in the morning as soon as your feet hit the floor. For some of you, this may work great, but for others, you may prefer the afternoon. Either way, just try to get some stretching into your routine at least three days a week. The Gazelle can also help with stretching. I always try to stretch for about five or ten minutes after I exercise. This helps relax the muscles and also helps you to cool down after your workout.

Chapter 6

Stand Up Tall and Sit Up Straight

We all know just how important it is to stand up tall and sit up straight, but for whatever reason, we chose not to. Standing up tall and sitting up straight is just as important as eating your vegetables every day! They are both habits necessary for optimal health. Standing up tall and sitting up straight is not only going to help your back but help strengthen those abs as well. When you stand up tall and sit up straight, you automatically pull in your stomach muscles. And by doing this all the time, you are going to work those abs. And if you add a few breathing exercise along with standing up tall and sitting up straight, you'll definitely burn a few calories … and all without sweating, if I might add! Go ahead and try it!

Forming this habit will be hard at first just like any other change we make in our lives, but just keep this in mind. You wouldn't go without brushing your teeth, would you? Stand up tall and sit up straight. It's that important. So please stand up tall and sit up straight!

If you are one of those individuals with back problems and can't really stand up tall or sit up straight, please give chiropractic therapy or acupuncture a try. They both can help with back problems and a lot of other health issues.

I've personally been seeing a chiropractor for about twelve years now. I started going when I was twenty-three years old. I had numbness in my right hip and leg. If I sat for longer than ten minutes anywhere, I would lose my balance when I would stand and sometimes fall. It sucked because I felt so young, but at the same time, I felt so old from the pain. I think it came from an epidural that I received when I was having my first child. The left side of my body went numb while my right side felt all the pain of childbirth. All the doctors said this was perfectly normal, but I felt and heard bones cracking like wine glasses hitting a tile floor. For two years, I went to doctor after doctor, and the only relief they could give me was pain medicine. Thanks but no thanks. I had given up hope and learned only to sit for short periods of time. That meant no movies for this chick of twenty-three unless I wanted to stand in the aisle at the movie theater. But God heard my cries and sent me a newspaper ad for a local chiropractor. I thought, *What did I have to lose?* The pain hopefully. And I did lose that pain forever! The chiropractor x-rayed me and asked questions just like any good doctor. He then adjusted my spine and aligned my hips. I even heard and felt a gigantic pop noise when he did my hips. The pressure from my hip was gone, I tell you! That night, I celebrated by taking my two-year-old to see *Winnie the Pooh* in the theater.

Now many years later, I not only go every two weeks, but I take my four children as well. My children will actually come to me and say, "Mommy, I really need to go to the chiropractor. I'm hurting here and here, and I fell today on the playground. Can we please go today or tomorrow? Mommy, you know only he can make it better. Please can we go?"

It's funny, but kids are very in tuned with their bodies, a lot more than us adults sometimes are. We adults just grin and bear all life's troubles. Kids feel pain and want the world to know it, which is a good thing. That's how they get it fixed. Smart creatures, aren't they? We adults could learn a lot from them, I think.

Chiropractic may not be your solution, but it doesn't hurt to try, because you just never know. It may the missing link to standing up tall and sitting up straight for you.

Acupuncture can also help with back problems as well as a lot of other health problems. I personally see an acupuncturist who is also a doctor of oriental medicine. She is a great addition to my well-being. Not only does she balance my yin and yang, but she also prescribes different herbs so that the body can heal itself naturally.

According to Chinese medicine, the yin and yang have to be balanced to allow the body to function properly. Sounds silly, I know, but when my yin and yang are imbalanced, I'm a very stressed-out person who feels like screaming at the world! But that's life, and life is stressful. It doesn't matter who you are, whether you are rich or poor, married or divorced, parent or not. If you are alive, you have stress! So my advice is to get your yin and yang balanced.

My oldest two children love acupuncture. My oldest daughter, who is fourteen years old, said that acupuncture gives her an inner peace like nothing else, not even her horse! That floored me, because this child is horse crazy. My son, who is now twelve years old, started acupuncture when he was six years old. He was diagnosed with a cancerous brain tumor called medulloblastoma. His doctor, who was from California, suggested we try acupuncture to relieve some of the pain from the chemo drugs. My son would cry for acupuncture. He said that it was the only thing that got rid of the pain! I would call her, and she would come and put needles all over his little body. Thirty minutes later, my son would be running around like a normal, happy, healthy six-year-old boy. I thank God every day for Dr. Mari Mengarelli and her needles!

After she would finish with my son, she always put a few needles in me. She would say, "You need this just as much as your son, honey. Your body is under a lot of stress from being a mom, especially a mom whose child is sick." Those needles gave me courage and strength. I needed that and still do to this day. Life is full of challenges, but you can handle life better if you're balanced!

When your body is constantly in stress mode, it will make you sick! That's why I do acupuncture to keep my body and mind balanced. Therefore, I'm less likely to get sick or have pain. I don't know about you, but I don't like being sick or having any type of pain.

Just like chiropractic therapy, acupuncture may not be for you, but it doesn't hurt to try something new, because you just never know. It may be just the answer you are looking for. As with all doctors research their credentials and ask family, friends, and coworkers for referrals to reputable practitioners with whom they may have had experience. Regarding acupuncturists, make sure they have a doctorate in acupuncture and Oriental medicine. That way, they can prescribe herbal formulas as well.

Good luck with whatever you choose! The important thing is to train yourself to sit up straight and stand up tall! Most of us don't do this. We slump over at our desks or the steering wheel and at home on the couch. Our spine is the foundation for our bodies. All our nerves meet at the spine. All messaging comes and goes from the spine. Standing up tall and sitting up straight is not only going to make you feel better but help you look better too. This is going to boost your self-esteem. This may sound silly or totally off the wall, but standing up tall and sitting up straight is going to boost your self-esteem. "Why?" you ask. Because you're going to feel better, and that's automatically going to make you look better and feel better about yourself. When you stand up tall and sit up straight, you work your abdominal muscles. No, it's not like doing a hundred sit-ups, but it will work your abs slowly. Add some breathing exercises in there, and you've got a mini workout. And for the women reading this, add some kegel exercises in as well, the ones where you squeeze the vagina muscles and count to ten and then release and repeat the process about ten times. They really do work! I tend to do these while I'm driving or sitting at my desk. You can also pull your stomach muscles in and out while you are breathing. This will work those abs, too.

And just think—you're still not sweating!

The important thing is to remember to stand up tall and sit up straight!

Chapter 7

Cutting Calories My Way

Here are some helpfully tips for cutting calories:
Eat your hamburger or sandwich with only one bun, especially if the bread is not high in fiber. You could save a hundred to two hundred calories. Choose mustard or very little mayo. The mayo alone can have anywhere from 150 to 250 calories.

With salads, lose the ranch and go for olive oil and vinegar. Ranch has 120 calories in two tablespoons. I know that I personally would use about eight tablespoons before! That's almost a thousand calories, and I haven't even added the cheese and croutons yet! When sprinkled on a salad, olive oil and vinegar will maybe add about 100 to 150 calories. Plus, olive oil is great for your digestive system.

Try a chai tea at Starbucks instead of those lattes. Chai tea has about 150 calories, and it's loaded with antioxidants. Go for the nonfat version! Some lattes can have as much as a thousand calories in them.

Go for grilled foods! One grilled chicken breast has about 100 to 150 calories. Get it fried, and you almost double the calories. Seafood is a great option if you choose grilled.

Cheese pizza has anywhere from three to four hundred calories per slice. I personally soak the top of my pizza with napkins. That takes off at least 150 calories in nothing but pure grease! It may sound weird. People may ask you what you are doing. Tell them you're saving your heart, because now all that grease is in the napkin and not your arteries!

If you choose to do the detox cleanse in chapter 4, please continue to drink the fiber and orange mix in the morning. Once you're done with the cleanse, you can keep drinking this every day for the rest of your life. At first, I didn't. Now I do. Trust me, this makes a huge difference! It beats eating or drinking prunes at the retirement home. And remember, it tastes great, and it's good for you. It'll keep your tummy and you happy!

For breakfast, try one of the Fiber One bars or pop one of the VitaTops in the toaster. They are both loaded in fiber and taste great too.

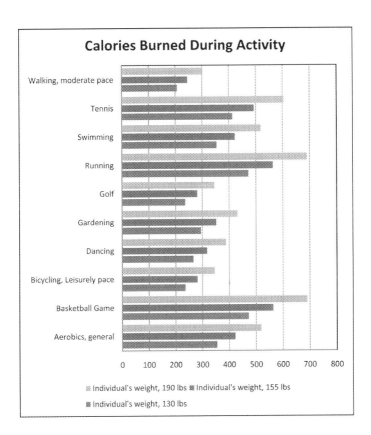

Calories Burned During Activity

Walking, moderate pace
Tennis
Swimming
Running
Golf
Gardening
Dancing
Bicycling, Leisurely pace
Basketball Game
Aerobics, general

0   100   200   300   400   500   600   700   800

■ Individual's weight, 190 lbs   ■ Individual's weight, 155 lbs
■ Individual's weight, 130 lbs

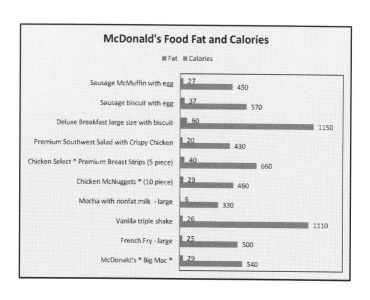

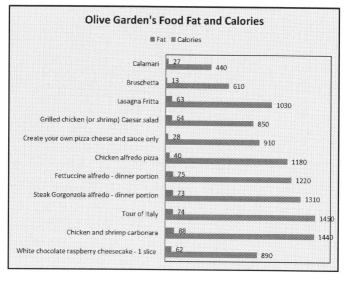

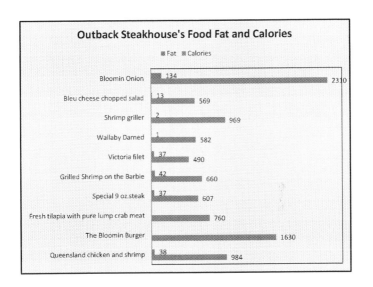

Outback Steakhouse's Food Fat and Calories

※ Fat ※ Calories

Food	Fat	Calories
Bloomin Onion	134	2310
Bleu cheese chopped salad	13	569
Shrimp griller	2	969
Wallaby Darned	1	582
Victoria filet	37	490
Grilled Shrimp on the Barbie	42	660
Special 9 oz.steak	37	607
Fresh tilapia with pure lump crab meat		760
The Bloomin Burger		1630
Queensland chicken and shrimp	38	984

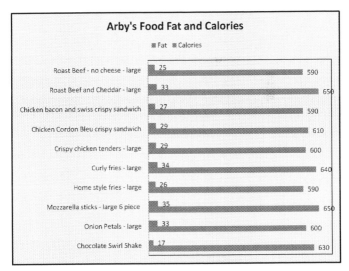

Arby's Food Fat and Calories

※ Fat ※ Calories

Food	Fat	Calories
Roast Beef - no cheese - large	25	590
Roast Beef and Cheddar - large	33	650
Chicken bacon and swiss crispy sandwich	27	590
Chicken Cordon Bleu crispy sandwich	29	610
Crispy chicken tenders - large	29	600
Curly fries - large	34	640
Home style fries - large	26	590
Mozzarella sticks - large 6 piece	35	650
Onion Petals - large	33	600
Chocolate Swirl Shake	17	630

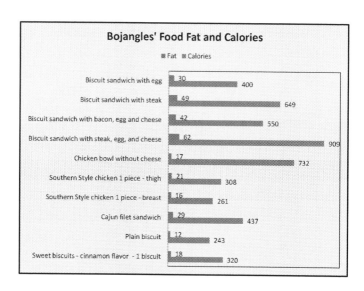

Bojangles' Food Fat and Calories

■ Fat ■ Calories

Biscuit sandwich with egg	30 / 400
Biscuit sandwich with steak	49 / 649
Biscuit sandwich with bacon, egg and cheese	42 / 550
Biscuit sandwich with steak, egg, and cheese	62 / 909
Chicken bowl without cheese	17 / 732
Southern Style chicken 1 piece - thigh	21 / 308
Southern Style chicken 1 piece - breast	16 / 261
Cajun filet sandwich	29 / 437
Plain biscuit	12 / 243
Sweet biscuits - cinnamon flavor - 1 biscuit	18 / 320

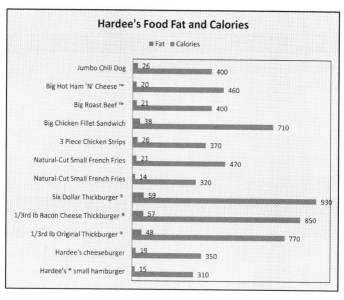

Hardee's Food Fat and Calories

■ Fat ■ Calories

Jumbo Chili Dog	26 / 400
Big Hot Ham 'N' Cheese ™	20 / 460
Big Roast Beef ™	21 / 400
Big Chicken Fillet Sandwich	38 / 710
3 Piece Chicken Strips	26 / 370
Natural-Cut Small French Fries	21 / 470
Natural-Cut Small French Fries	14 / 320
Six Dollar Thickburger ®	59 / 930
1/3rd lb Bacon Cheese Thickburger ®	57 / 850
1/3rd lb Original Thickburger ®	48 / 770
Hardee's cheeseburger	19 / 350
Hardee's ® small hamburger	15 / 310

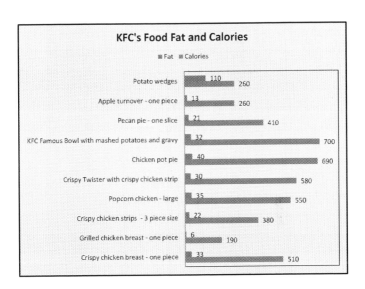

KFC's Food Fat and Calories

■ Fat ■ Calories

Food	Fat	Calories
Potato wedges	110	260
Apple turnover - one piece	13	260
Pecan pie - one slice	21	410
KFC Famous Bowl with mashed potatoes and gravy	32	700
Chicken pot pie	40	690
Crispy Twister with crispy chicken strip	30	580
Popcorn chicken - large	35	550
Crispy chicken strips - 3 piece size	22	380
Grilled chicken breast - one piece	6	190
Crispy chicken breast - one piece	33	510

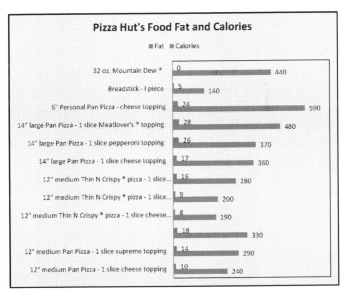

Pizza Hut's Food Fat and Calories

■ Fat ■ Calories

Food	Fat	Calories
32 oz. Mountain Dew *	0	440
Breadstick - I piece	5	140
6" Personal Pan Pizza - cheese topping	24	590
14" large Pan Pizza - 1 slice Meatlover's * topping	28	480
14" large Pan Pizza - 1 slice pepperoni topping	26	370
14" large Pan Pizza - 1 slice cheese topping	17	360
12" medium Thin N Crispy * pizza - 1 slice...	16	280
12" medium Thin N Crispy * pizza - 1 slice...	9	200
12" medium Thin N Crispy * pizza - 1 slice cheese...	8	190
	18	330
12" medium Pan Pizza - 1 slice supreme topping	14	290
12" medium Pan Pizza - 1 slice cheese topping	10	240

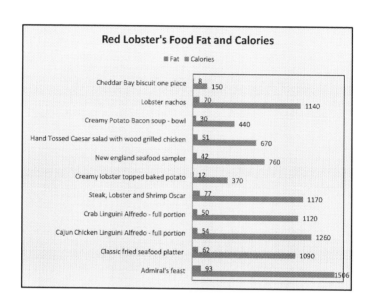

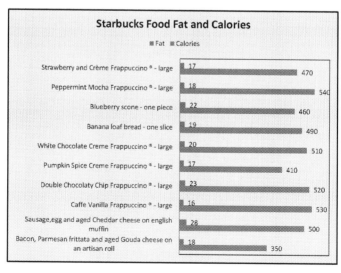

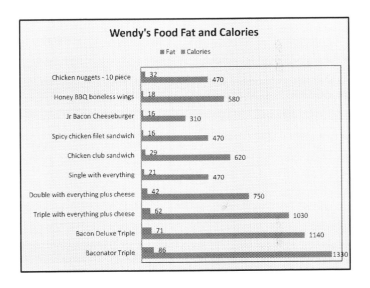

Journal:

About The Author

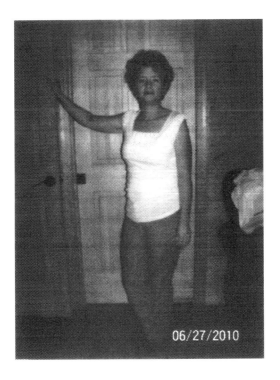

06/27/2010

This book was written for the sole purpose of helping people like me who have battled with wanting weight loss. All information in this book is based on my own personal experience with wanting to lose weight and be healthy!

Printed in the United States
By Bookmasters